MW01137350

Makeup Tutorial for Teens and Beginners:

Tricks and Tips How to Make Ideal
Makeup

Description

Welcome to "Makeup Tutorial Book for Teens and Beginners: Tricks and Tips How to Make Ideal Makeup"! In this eBook, you'll find everything you need to know to create beautiful, flawless makeup looks that enhance your natural beauty.

From choosing the right products and tools, to learning different techniques and makeup styles, this eBook is packed with valuable information and tips to help you master the art of makeup. Whether you're a beginner or an experienced makeup user, you'll find something to help you create looks that are flattering, wearable, and appropriate for any occasion.

With chapters on skincare, foundation, eyes, lips, and more, this eBook is a comprehensive guide to all things makeup. So let's get started and learn how to create the perfect makeup look!

Following points have been discussed in this eBook:

- Introduction to makeup
- Choosing the right products
- Skincare routine before makeup
- Foundation and concealer techniques
- Contouring and highlighting
- Eye makeup techniques (e.g., eyeshadow, eyeliner, mascara)
- Lip makeup techniques (e.g., lip liner, lipstick)
- Blush and bronzer application
- Makeup for different occasions (e.g., everyday makeup, evening makeup, special event makeup)
- Makeup for different face shapes
- Makeup for different skin tones
- Makeup for different eye shapes
- Makeup for different lip shapes
- Makeup for different brow shapes
- Makeup for different hair colors

- Makeup for different age groups (e.g., teenage makeup, mature makeup)
- Makeup trends and looks
- Makeup removal and skincare routine after makeup
- Makeup storage and organization
- Bonus tips and tricks for achieving the perfect makeup look
- Ten Steps Guide to Perfect Makeup
- Special Makeup Applications
- Skin secrets
- Conclusion

Once you will buy this book, you will keep on checking this guide for quick tricks, guidance, and easy-to-follow instructions again and again. So, what are you waiting for? Start your journey today!

TABLE OF CONTENTS

Introduction

Welcome to your makeup tutorial book! In this book, we'll be covering a range of topics to help you master the art of makeup and achieve the perfect look. Whether you're a beginner or a seasoned pro, you'll find something new and useful in these pages.

In this first chapter, we'll start by introducing the world of makeup and its history. Makeup has been around for thousands of years, and it's evolved significantly over time. In ancient civilizations, makeup was often used to indicate social status or religious beliefs. In modern times, makeup is used for a variety of purposes, including enhancing natural beauty, expressing personal style, and boosting confidence.

In this book, we'll be focusing on makeup for teens and beginners. We'll cover the basics of choosing the right products, applying makeup correctly, and creating different looks for different occasions. We'll also delve into more advanced techniques, such as contouring and highlighting, and discuss how to customize your makeup routine based on your unique features and preferences.

So let's get started on your makeup journey! Whether you're looking to try out a new look or just want to improve your everyday makeup routine, this book has something for you.

Chapter 1: Choosing the right products

When it comes to makeup, the right products can make all the difference. Choosing the right products means finding ones that suit your skin type and concerns, as well as your personal style and preferences. In this chapter, we'll discuss how to select the best products for you.

<u>Understanding product formulations and ingredients</u>

One of the first things to consider when choosing makeup products is the formulation. Different types of products (e.g., foundation, lipstick, eyeshadow) have different formulations, and it's important to choose one that will work well with your skin. For example, if you have oily skin, you may want to opt for a matte foundation rather than a dewy one. If you have sensitive skin, you may want to avoid products with certain ingredients (e.g., alcohol, fragrances) that can cause irritation.

It's also important to pay attention to the ingredients in your makeup products. Some ingredients can be beneficial for your skin (e.g., antioxidants, vitamins), while others can be harmful or irritating (e.g. sulfates, parabens). Read the ingredient list carefully and do some research to understand the benefits and drawbacks of each ingredient.

SELECTING PRODUCTS BASED ON SKIN TYPE AND CONCERNS

In addition to the formulation, it's important to choose makeup products that are suitable for your skin type. Different products are formulated for different skin types (e.g., dry, oily, combination, sensitive), and using the wrong products can lead to problems such as dryness, breakouts, or an uneven finish.

You should also consider any specific skin concerns you may have when choosing makeup products. For example, if you have acne-prone skin, you may want to choose oil-free or non-comedogenic products to avoid clogging pores. If you have dark circles or uneven skin tone, you may want to look for products with color-correcting or brightening properties.

Choosing the right tools

In addition to the products themselves, it's important to choose the right tools to apply your makeup. Makeup brushes, sponges, and other tools can make a big difference in the way your makeup looks and how easy it is to apply.

When choosing makeup brushes, look for ones that are made of high-quality materials (e.g., synthetic fibers, natural hairs) and are appropriate for the type of product you're using. For example, a dense, flat brush is good for packing on eyeshadow, while a fluffy, dome-shaped brush is good for blending.

Makeup sponges can also be useful tools, particularly for applying liquid or cream products. Look for sponges that are soft, bouncy, and easy to clean.

With the right products and tools, you'll be well on your way to achieving perfect makeup looks!

Chapter 2: Skincare routine before makeup

Before you start applying makeup, it's important to have a good skincare routine in place. Taking care of your skin will not only help your makeup look better, but it will also improve the overall health and appearance of your skin. In this chapter, we'll discuss the steps you should take before applying makeup.

Cleansing and toning

The first step in your skincare routine should be cleansing and toning. Cleansing removes dirt, oil, and other impurities from the skin, while toning helps to balance the pH of the skin and prepare it for the next steps in your routine.

To cleanse your skin, use a gentle cleanser that is suitable for your skin type. Apply the cleanser to your face and neck, using circular motions to massage it in. Rinse the cleanser off with lukewarm water, then pat your skin dry with a clean towel.

After cleansing, you can follow up with a toner. Toner can help to remove any remaining impurities, as well as tighten and tone the skin. Simply apply the toner to a cotton pad and swipe it over your face and neck.

Applying moisturizer and/or primer

The next step in your skincare routine should be moisturizing. Moisturizer helps to hydrate the skin and keep it looking plump and healthy. Choose a moisturizer that is suitable for your skin type and any specific concerns you may have (e.g., acne-prone, mature).

In addition to moisturizer, you may also want to use a primer before applying makeup. Primer helps to smooth out the texture of the skin and create a smooth canvas for your makeup. It can also help to extend the wear of your makeup and prevent it from creasing or smudging.

Treating specific skin concerns

If you have specific skin concerns (e.g. acne, dark spots), you may want to incorporate additional steps into your skincare routine. For example, you may want to use a spot treatment to target acne, or a serum with brightening ingredients to fade dark spots. Consult with a dermatologist or a skincare professional if you have severe or persistent skin concerns.

By following a good skincare routine before applying makeup, you'll be starting with a clean, healthy canvas that will help your makeup look its best.

Chapter 3: Foundation and concealer techniques

Foundation and concealer are the building blocks of a good makeup look. They help to even out the skin tone and create a smooth, cohesive base for the rest of your makeup. In this chapter, we'll cover the basics of applying foundation and concealer correctly.

Finding the right shade of foundation

Finding the right shade of foundation is crucial to achieving a natural, seamless finish. Your foundation should match your skin tone as closely as possible, without being too light or too dark.

To find the right shade of foundation, test a few shades on your jawline, rather than the back of your hand. This will give you a better idea of how the color looks on your face. You can also ask for a sample of a foundation before purchasing a full-size bottle to make sure it's a good match.

Applying foundation with a brush, sponge, or fingers

There are several ways to apply foundation, and the best method for you will depend on your personal preference and the type of foundation you're using. Here are some options:

- Brush: A makeup brush can be used to apply liquid or powder foundation. Look for a brush with synthetic fibers that are densely packed and soft.

- Sponge: A makeup sponge (e.g. Beauty blender) can be used to apply liquid or cream foundation. Dampen the sponge slightly before using it to help the foundation blend seamlessly into the skin.

- Fingers: You can also apply foundation with your fingers, particularly if you're using a cream or stick foundation. Simply dot the foundation onto your skin and blend it in using circular motions.

Whichever method you choose, be sure to blend the foundation well to avoid streaks or lines.

Using concealer to cover blemishes, dark circles, and redness

Concealer is a versatile product that can be used to cover a variety of imperfections, including blemishes, dark circles, and redness. When applying concealer, it's important to choose the right shade and formula for your needs.

To cover blemishes, use a concealer that is slightly lighter than your skin tone and has good coverage. Apply the concealer directly to the blemish, then blend it out using a brush or sponge.

To cover dark circles, use a concealer that is one shade lighter than your skin tone and has a brightening effect. Apply the concealer under your eyes, starting at the inner corner and blending outward.

To cover redness, use a concealer that is green toned to neutralize the redness. Apply the concealer to the red areas, then blend it out using a brush or sponge.

By using foundation and concealer correctly, you can create a smooth, even base for the rest of your makeup.

Chapter 4: Contouring and highlighting

Contouring and highlighting are techniques that can be used to add dimension and shape to the face. By using different shades of makeup, you can create the illusion of shadows and light, and enhance or alter the natural contours of your face. In this chapter, we'll cover the basics of contouring and highlighting.

Understanding the basics of facial contouring

Contouring involves using a darker shade of makeup to create shadows on the face, while highlighting involves using a lighter shade to create highlights. When done correctly, contouring and highlighting can help to define and sculpt the features of the face, creating the illusion of a more chiseled or defined look.

To contour, you'll need a matte, neutral-toned product that is one to two shades darker than your skin tone. To highlight, you'll need a shimmery or iridescent product that is one to two shades lighter than your skin tone. You can use a variety of products for contouring and highlighting, including powder, cream, or liquid products.

Choosing the right contour shades for your skin tone

When choosing contour shades, it's important to consider your skin tone. If you have a fair to medium skin tone, look for contour shades that are in the taupe or ash brown range. If you have a medium to deep skin tone, look for contour shades that are in the chestnut or deep brown range. Avoid contour shades that are too orange or red, as these can look unnatural.

Applying contour and highlight products

To apply contour and highlight products, start by identifying the areas of your face that you want to define or enhance. Common areas to contour include the sides of the nose, the hollows of the cheeks, and the jawline. Common areas to highlight include the brow bone, the inner corners of the eyes, the center of the nose, and the Cupid's bow.

Using a brush or sponge, apply the contour product to the areas you want to define, blending it out well to avoid harsh lines. Then, apply the highlight product to the areas you want to enhance, blending it out in a circular motion.

Contouring and highlighting can take some practice to get right, so don't be afraid to experiment and see what works best for you. With a little bit of practice, you'll be able to create a natural-looking dimension and shape on your face.

Chapter 5: Eye makeup techniques

Eyes are often the focus of a makeup look, and there are endless ways to enhance and play up your eye makeup. In this chapter, we'll cover some basic techniques for applying eyeshadow, eyeliner, and mascara.

Applying eyeshadow

Eyeshadow can be used to add color, depth, and dimension to the eyes. There are countless eyeshadow shades and formulas to choose from, ranging from matte to shimmery, neutral to bold.

To apply eyeshadow, start by selecting a color palette that complements your eye color and the overall look you're going for. Then, use a brush to apply the eyeshadow to your lid, blending it out well to avoid harsh lines. You can also use a lighter shade on the inner corner of the eye and a darker shade in the crease to add depth and dimension.

Some popular eyeshadow looks include:

- Neutral eyeshadow: A neutral eyeshadow look is perfect for everyday wear or a more subtle, natural look. Use a palette of beige, taupe, and brown shades to create a seamless, effortless look.

- Smoky eye: A smoky eye is a classic look that involves using darker, more intense shades of eyeshadow to create a smudged, sultry effect.

To create a smoky eye, use a brush or sponge to apply a dark shade of eyes.

Chapter 6: Eyeliner techniques

Eyeliner is a versatile product that can be used to enhance the shape and definition of the eyes. There are several types of eyeliner to choose from, including pencil, liquid, and gel, and each type has its own unique properties and application techniques. In this chapter, we'll cover some basic techniques for applying eyeliner.

Pencil eyeliner

Pencil eyeliner is a classic and easy-to-use option. It comes in a solid form that can be sharpened to a fine point for precise application. Pencil eyeliner can be used to create a variety of looks, from a thin, subtle line to a bold, dramatic cat eye.

To apply pencil eyeliner, start by pulling the skin around your eye taut. Then, use short, feathery strokes to line your upper and lower lashes. If you're going for a more precise line, you can use a ruler or a business card to guide your hand. To smudge the liner for a softer, more diffused look, use a brush or your finger to blend it out.

Liquid eyeliner

Liquid eyeliner is a more precise and longer-lasting option, but it can be more challenging to apply. It comes in a liquid form that is applied with a brush or a felt-tip pen. Liquid eyeliner is ideal for creating precise lines, including thin, classic lines and bold, dramatic cat eyes.

To apply liquid eyeliner, start by pulling the skin around your eye taut. Then, use a steady hand to draw a line along your upper lashes, starting at the inner corner of the eye and working outward. If you're going for a more dramatic cat eye, extend the line beyond the outer corner of the eye and flick it upward. To create a winged look, draw a line from the outer corner of the eye to the end of the brow bone.

Gel eyeliner

Gel eyeliner is a creamy, long-lasting option that is applied with a brush. It is similar to liquid eyeliner in terms of precision and staying power, but it is easier to control and can be smudged for a softer, more diffused look. Gel eyeliner is ideal for creating a variety of looks, from thin, classic lines to bold, dramatic wings.

To apply gel eyeliner, start by pulling the skin around your eye taut. Then, use a brush to draw a line along your upper lashes, starting at the inner corner of the eye and working outward. If you're going for a more dramatic cat eye or winged look, extend the line beyond the outer corner of the eye and flick it upward. To create a smudged, sultry look, use the brush to blend the liner out along the upper and lower lashes.

By mastering different eyeliner techniques, you'll be able to create a wide range of looks and add definition and drama to your eyes.

Chapter 7: Mascara techniques

Mascara is a makeup staple that can help to lengthen, thicken, and define your lashes. There are many types of mascara to choose from, including volumizing, lengthening, and curling, and each type has its own unique properties and application techniques. In this chapter, we'll cover some basic techniques for applying mascara.

Choosing the right mascara for your lashes

Before you apply mascara, it's important to choose the right formula for your lashes. If you have short, thin lashes, you may want to opt for a volumizing mascara that will add thickness and fullness to your lashes. If you have long, straight lashes, you may want to try a lengthening mascara that will add length and separation to your lashes. If you have naturally curly lashes, you may want to try a curling mascara that will help to enhance and define your curl.

Applying mascara

To apply mascara, start by wiggling the brush at the base of your lashes to deposit the product. Then, use a zig-zag motion to work the mascara through the length of your lashes. Be sure to coat both the top and bottom lashes for a full and defined look.

If you're using a volumizing mascara, you may want to apply a few extra coats to build up the volume and fullness of your lashes. If you're using a lengthening mascara, you may want to use a brush with long, fine bristles to separate and lengthen your lashes. If you're using a curling mascara, you may want to use a brush with a curved shape to help lift and curl your lashes.

Removing mascara

To remove mascara, use a gentle eye makeup remover or a mild, oil-based cleanser. Dab a small amount of the product onto a cotton pad, then gently swipe it over your lashes to dissolve the mascara. Be sure to remove all traces of mascara, as leaving it on overnight can lead to clumps and flakes.

By mastering different mascara techniques, you'll be able to enhance and define your lashes to suit your desired look. Whether you want long, luscious lashes or full, voluminous ones, a good mascara can make a big difference in your overall makeup look.

Chapter 8: Lip makeup techniques

Lip makeup is a fun and easy way to add color and dimension to your look. There are many types of lip products to choose from, including lipstick, lip gloss, and lip liner, and each type has its own unique properties and application techniques. In this chapter, we'll cover some basic techniques for applying lip makeup.

Choosing the right lip product for your desired look

Before you apply lip makeup, it's important to choose the right product for your desired look. If you want a bold, long-lasting color, you may want to opt for a lipstick. If you want a glossy, moisturizing finish, you may want to try a lip gloss. If you want precise, defined lips, you may want to use a lip liner.

Applying lipstick

To apply lipstick, start by exfoliating your lips to remove any dry, flaky skin. Then, line your lips with a lip liner to help define the shape and prevent the lipstick from feathering. Finally, apply the lipstick to your lips, starting at the center and working outward. Be sure to blend the edges well to avoid harsh lines.

If you're using a bold or dark shade of lipstick, you may want to use a lip brush to apply the product for more precise application. You can also blot your lips with a tissue to remove excess product and create a matte finish.

Applying lip gloss

To apply lip gloss, start by applying a lip balm or a lip primer to moisturize and prep your lips. Then, apply the lip gloss to your lips, starting at the center and working outward. For a more precise application, you can use a lip brush.

If you want to create a gradient lip look, you can apply a lighter shade of gloss to the center of your lips and a darker shade to the outer edges. You can also layer different shades of gloss to create a customized color.

Applying lip liner

To apply lip liner, start by outlining your natural lip line, following the shape of your lips. Then, fill in your lips with the lip liner, blending it well to avoid harsh lines.

Lip liner can be used to define and shape the lips, as well as to prevent lipstick from feathering or bleeding. You can use a lip liner that is the same shade as your lipstick for a seamless look, or you can mix and match shades to create a customized color.

By mastering different lip makeup techniques, you'll be able to create a wide range of looks and add color and dimension to your lips. Whether you want a bold, statement lip or a subtle, natural one, the right lip makeup can help you achieve your desired look.

Chapter 9: Makeup for different occasions

Makeup looks can vary widely depending on the occasion. A dramatic, smokey eye may be perfect for a night out, but may be too intense for a more casual, daytime event. In this chapter, we'll cover some basic guidelines for selecting the right makeup for different occasions.

Makeup for everyday wear

For everyday wear, you'll want to choose makeup that is natural and easy to wear. Look for products that are lightweight and buildable, so you can create a subtle, effortless look. Some key products to consider for everyday wear include:

- Tinted moisturizer or BB cream: These lightweight, multi-tasking products provide light coverage and hydration, while also evening out the skin tone.

- Mascara: A few coats of mascara can help to define and lengthen your lashes, without looking too heavy or over-the-top.

- Lip balm or lip gloss: A moisturizing lip product can help to keep your lips hydrated and looking healthy, without being too bold or distracting.

Makeup for special occasions

For special occasions, you may want to go a bit more glam with your makeup look. Look for products that are long-lasting and have a more dramatic effect, such as:

- Full-coverage foundation: A full-coverage foundation can help to create a flawless, airbrushed effect, and will stay put through the duration of your event.

- Bold eyeshadow: A bold eyeshadow shade can add drama and impact to your look. Look for a shimmery or metallic shade to really make your eyes pop.

- Dramatic eyeliner: Whether it's a bold, winged cat eye or a thick, smudgy line, dramatic eyeliner can help to make a statement with your eye makeup.

- Long-lasting lipstick: For a lip look that will last through the night, opt for a long-wearing lipstick formula. Matte lipsticks tend to be more long-lasting, but there are also many hydrating, long-wearing formulas available.

By considering the occasion and the desired effect, you'll be able to choose the right makeup products and techniques to create a look that is appropriate and flattering.

Makeup for professional settings

In a professional setting, it's important to choose makeup that is subtle, polished, and appropriate for the workplace. Look for products that are natural and understated, such as:

- Tinted moisturizer or BB cream: A lightweight, sheer coverage product can help

to even out the skin tone and create a natural, healthy-looking glow.

- Mascara: A few coats of mascara can help to define and lengthen your lashes, without looking too heavy or over-the-top.

- Lip balm or lipstick: Choose a subtle, natural-looking shade of lip product that is moisturizing and polished. Avoid bold or glossy shades, as these can be distracting in a professional setting.

By following these guidelines, you'll be able to create a makeup look that is appropriate and professional in any setting.

Chapter 10: Makeup for different skin tones

Makeup looks can vary widely depending on your skin tone. Different shades and tones of makeup will look different on different skin tones, and it's important to choose products that complement your natural coloring. In this chapter, we'll cover some

basic guidelines for selecting makeup for different skin tones.

Makeup for fair skin tones

If you have a fair skin tone, you'll want to choose makeup that is light and subtle, so as not to overpower your natural coloring. Look for products that are sheer and luminous, such as:

- Tinted moisturizer or BB cream: A sheer, lightweight formula will help to even out your skin tone without looking heavy or cakey.

- Soft, neutral eyeshadow: A neutral eyeshadow palette will help to enhance your natural eye color and create a subtle, effortless look.

- Light, natural lipstick: Choose a light, natural shade of lipstick that is moisturizing and enhances your natural lip color.

Makeup for medium skin tones

If you have a medium skin tone, you'll have a bit more flexibility with your makeup choices. Look for products that are medium in coverage and intensity, such as:

- Medium-coverage foundation: A medium-coverage foundation will help to even out your skin tone and provide a natural, luminous finish.

- Bold eyeshadow: A bold eyeshadow shade can add drama and impact to your look. Look for a shimmery or metallic shade to really make your eyes pop.

- Bold lipstick: A bold lipstick shade can add a pop of color to your look. Look for a shade that complements your skin tone and enhances your natural lip color.

Makeup for dark skin tones

If you have a dark skin tone, you'll want to choose makeup that is rich and vibrant, to complement your

natural coloring. Look for products that are highly pigmented and have a strong color payoff, such as:

- Full-coverage foundation: A full-coverage foundation will help to even out your skin tone and provide a flawless, airbrushed effect.

- Vibrant eyeshadow: A vibrant eyeshadow shade can add drama and impact to your look. Look for a shimmery or metallic shade to really make your eyes pop.

- Vibrant lipstick: A vibrant lipstick shade can add a pop of color to your look. Look for a shade that complements your skin tone and enhances your natural lip color.

By considering your skin tone and selecting makeup that complements your natural coloring, you'll be able to create a look that is flattering and enhances your natural beauty.

Chapter 11: Makeup for different eye shapes

Makeup looks can vary widely depending on the shape of your eyes. Different techniques and products will help to enhance and balance different eye shapes. In this chapter, we'll cover some basic guidelines for selecting makeup for different eye shapes.

Makeup for almond-shaped eyes

If you have almond-shaped eyes, you're lucky, as this is considered the ideal eye shape. Almond-shaped eyes are balanced and symmetrical, with a natural upward slope at the outer corners. To enhance this eye shape, you'll want to focus on creating a smoky, diffused look, using a combination of light and dark shades:

- Light eyeshadow: Apply a light, shimmery eyeshadow to the inner corners of the eyes and the brow bone to brighten and open up the eyes.

- Dark eyeshadow: Use a dark, matte eyeshadow to define the crease and outer corner of the eyes, creating a smoky, diffused effect.

- Eyeliner: Use a soft, smudgy eyeliner to line the upper and lower lashes, blending it well for a seamless, smoky effect.

Makeup for round eyes

If you have round eyes, you'll want to focus on creating a more elongated, almond-shaped look. To do this, you'll want to use techniques that lift and elongate the eyes, such as:

- Light eyeshadow: Apply a light, shimmery eyeshadow to the inner corners of the eyes and the brow bone to brighten and open up the eyes.

- Dark eyeshadow: Use a dark, matte eyeshadow to define the outer corners of the eyes, creating a lifted, elongated effect.

- Eyeliner: Use a thin, precise eyeliner to line the upper lashes, extending the line slightly beyond the outer corners of the eyes to create a winged effect.

Makeup for hooded eyes

If you have hooded eyes, you'll want to focus on creating an open, defined eye shape. To do this, you'll want to use techniques that lift and open up the eyes, such as:

- Light eyeshadow: Apply a light, shimmery eyeshadow to the inner corners of the eyes and the brow bone to brighten and open up the eyes.

- Dark eyeshadow: Use a dark, matte eyeshadow to define the crease and outer corner of the eyes, creating a lifted, defined effect.

- Eyeliner: Use a thin, precise eyeliner to line the upper lashes, extending the line slightly beyond the outer corners of the eyes to create a winged effect. Avoid lining the lower lashes, as this can close off the eyes and create a heavy, droopy look.

By considering the shape of your eyes and using makeup techniques that enhance and balance your eye shape, you'll be able to create a look that is flattering and enhances the natural beauty of your eyes.

Makeup for small eyes

If you have small eyes, you'll want to focus on creating a more open, defined eye shape. To do this, you'll want to use techniques that open up and enlarge the eyes, such as:

- Light eyeshadow: Apply a light, shimmery eyeshadow to the inner corners of the eyes and the brow bone to brighten and open up the eyes.

- Dark eyeshadow: Use a dark, matte eyeshadow to define the crease and outer corner of the eyes, creating a lifted, defined effect.

- Eyeliner: Use a thin, precise eyeliner to line the upper lashes, extending the line slightly beyond the outer corners of the eyes to create a winged effect. Avoid lining the lower lashes, as this can close off the eyes and create a heavy, droopy look.

- Mascara: Use a lengthening mascara to add length and separation to your lashes, helping to open up and enlarge the eyes.

By using these techniques, you'll be able to create a look that enhances the natural beauty of your small eyes.

Chapter 12: Makeup for different face shapes

Makeup looks can vary widely depending on the shape of your face. Different techniques and products will help to balance and flatter different face shapes. In this chapter, we'll cover some basic guidelines for selecting makeup for different face shapes.

Makeup for round faces

If you have a round face, you'll want to focus on creating a more angular, elongated look. To do this, you'll want to use techniques that add definition and length to the face, such as:

- Contouring: Use a contouring product to define the cheekbones and jawline, creating a more angular, structured look.

- Highlighting: Use a highlighting product to bring light to the high points of the face, such as the brow bone and the center of the nose, to create a more elongated, slender effect.

- Winged eyeliner: Use a winged eyeliner technique to elongate and lift the eyes, helping to balance out the roundness of the face.

Makeup for oval faces

If you have an oval face, you're lucky, as this is considered the ideal face shape. Oval faces are balanced and symmetrical, with a natural narrowing at the jawline. To enhance this face shape, you can experiment with a wide range of makeup looks and techniques, as most will flatter your natural bone structure.

Makeup for square faces

If you have a square face, you'll want to focus on softening and balancing the angular lines of your face. To do this, you'll want to use techniques that add curves and roundness to the face, such as:

- Contouring: Use a contouring product to define the cheekbones and jawline, creating a more angular, structured look. Avoid contouring the jawline too heavily, as this can accentuate the squareness of the face.

- Highlighting: Use a highlighting product to bring light to the high points of the face, such as the brow bone and the center of the nose, to create a softer, more rounded effect.

- Soft, rounded eyebrows: Use a brow pencil or brow powder to shape and define your eyebrows, using a soft, rounded technique to create a more feminine, curved effect.

By considering the shape of your face and using makeup techniques that balance and flatter your features, you'll be able to create a look that enhances the natural beauty of your face.

Chapter 13: Makeup for different hair colors

Makeup looks can vary widely depending on your hair color. Different shades and tones of makeup will look different on different hair colors, and it's important to choose products that complement your natural coloring. In this chapter, we'll cover some basic guidelines for selecting makeup for different hair colors.

Makeup for blonde hair

If you have blonde hair, you'll want to choose makeup that is light and subtle, to complement your fair coloring. Look for products that are sheer and luminous, such as:

- Tinted moisturizer or BB cream: A sheer, lightweight formula will help to even out your skin tone without looking heavy or cakey.

- Soft, neutral eyeshadow: A neutral eyeshadow palette will help to enhance your natural eye color and create a subtle, effortless look.

- Light, natural lipstick: Choose a light, natural shade of lipstick that is moisturizing and enhances your natural lip color.

Makeup for brunette hair

If you have brunette hair, you'll have a bit more flexibility with your makeup choices. Look for products that are medium in coverage and intensity, such as:

- Medium-coverage foundation: A medium-coverage foundation will help to even out your skin tone and provide a natural, luminous finish.

- Bold eyeshadow: A bold eyeshadow shade can add drama and impact to your look. Look for a shimmery or metallic shade to really make your eyes pop.

- Bold lipstick: A bold lipstick shade can add a pop of color to your look. Look for a shade that complements your skin tone and enhances your natural lip color.

Makeup for red hair

If you have red hair, you'll want to choose makeup that is rich and vibrant, to complement your bold coloring. Look for products that are highly pigmented and have a strong color payoff, such as:

- Full-coverage foundation: A full-coverage foundation will help to even out your skin tone and provide a flawless, airbrushed effect.

- Vibrant eyeshadow: A vibrant eyeshadow shade can add drama and impact to your look. Look for a shimmery or metallic shade to really make your eyes pop.

- Vibrant lipstick: A vibrant lipstick shade can add a pop of color to your look. Look for a shade that complements your skin tone and enhances your natural lip color.

By considering your hair color and selecting makeup that complements your natural coloring, you'll be able to create a look that is flattering and enhances your natural beauty.

Chapter 14: Makeup for different age ranges

As we age, our skin and features change, and our makeup needs may also change. In this chapter, we'll cover some basic guidelines for selecting makeup for different age ranges.

Makeup for teens

If you're a teenager, you may be just starting to experiment with makeup. It's important to choose products that are age-appropriate and enhance your natural beauty. Look for products that are lightweight and natural-looking, such as:

- Tinted moisturizer or BB cream: A lightweight, sheer coverage product can help to even out your skin tone and create a natural, healthy-looking glow.

- Mascara: A few coats of mascara can help to define and lengthen your lashes, without looking too heavy or over-the-top.

- Lip balm or lipstick: Choose a subtle, natural-looking shade of lip product that is moisturizing and polished. Avoid bold or glossy shades, as these can be overwhelming for a youthful look.

Makeup for women in their 20s and 30s

If you're in your 20s or 30s, you may be more comfortable and confident with your makeup routine. At this age, you can experiment with a wider range of products and techniques, but it's still important to choose products that are appropriate for your skin type and concerns. Look for products that are hydrating and nourishing, such as:

- Foundation: Choose a foundation that is suitable for your skin type and provides the level of coverage you desire. Look for formulas that contain skin-loving ingredients, such as antioxidants and hyaluronic acid.

- Eyeshadow: Experiment with a range of eyeshadow shades and finishes, from neutral to bold. Look for long-wearing formulas that will stay put all day.

- Lipstick: Choose a lipstick that is moisturizing and comfortable to wear. Look for formulas that contain nourishing ingredients, such as shea butter and vitamin E.

Makeup for women in their 40s and beyond

As we age, our skin may become drier and more prone to fine lines and wrinkles. It's important to choose makeup products that are nourishing and hydrating, to help maintain the health and vitality of the skin. Look for products that are formulated for mature skin, such as:

- Foundation: Choose a foundation that is suitable for your skin type and provides the level of coverage you desire. Look for formulas that contain skin-loving ingredients, such as antioxidants and hyaluronic acid. Avoid matte formulas, as these can be drying and accentuate the appearance of fine lines and wrinkles.

- Eyeshadow: Experiment with a range of eyeshadow shades and finishes, from neutral to bold. Look for long-wearing formulas that will stay put all day. Avoid heavy, cakey formulas that can crease and settle into fine lines.

- Lipstick: Choose a lipstick that is moisturizing and comfortable to wear. Look for formulas that contain nourishing ingredients, such as shea butter and vitamin E. Avoid matte formulas, as these can be drying and accentuate the appearance of fine lines and wrinkles.

By choosing makeup products that are suitable for your age range and skin concerns, you'll be able to create a look that is flattering and enhances your natural beauty.

Chapter 15: Makeup for different skin tones

Makeup looks can vary widely depending on your skin tone. Different shades and tones of makeup will look different on different skin tones, and it's important to choose products that complement your natural coloring. In this chapter, we'll cover some basic guidelines for selecting makeup for different skin tones.

Makeup for fair skin

If you have fair skin, you'll want to choose makeup that is light and subtle, to complement your light coloring. Look for products that are sheer and luminous, such as:

- Tinted moisturizer or BB cream: A sheer, lightweight formula will help to even out your skin tone without looking heavy or cakey.

- Soft, neutral eyeshadow: A neutral eyeshadow palette will help to enhance your natural eye color and create a subtle, effortless look.

- Light, natural lipstick: Choose a light, natural shade of lipstick that is moisturizing and enhances your natural lip color.

Makeup for medium skin

If you have medium skin, you'll have a bit more flexibility with your makeup choices. Look for products that are medium in coverage and intensity, such as:

- Medium-coverage foundation: A medium-coverage foundation will help to even out your skin tone and provide a natural, luminous finish.

- Bold eyeshadow: A bold eyeshadow shade can add drama and impact to your look. Look for a shimmery or metallic shade to really make your eyes pop.

- Bold lipstick: A bold lipstick shade can add a pop of color to your look. Look for a shade that complements your skin tone and enhances your natural lip color.

Makeup for dark skin

If you have dark skin, you'll want to choose makeup that is rich and vibrant, to complement your bold coloring. Look for products that are highly pigmented and have a strong color payoff, such as:

- Full-coverage foundation: A full-coverage foundation will help to even out your skin tone and provide a flawless, airbrushed effect.

- Vibrant eyeshadow: A vibrant eyeshadow shade can add drama and impact to your look. Look for a shimmery or metallic shade to really make your eyes pop.

- Vibrant lipstick: A vibrant lipstick shade can add a pop of color to your look. Look for a shade that complements your skin tone and enhances your natural lip color.

By considering your skin tone and selecting makeup that complements your natural coloring, you'll be able to create a look that is flattering and enhances your natural beauty.

Chapter 16: Makeup for different skin types

Makeup looks can vary widely depending on your skin type. Different formulas and textures of makeup will work better on different skin types, and it's important to choose products that are suitable for your specific skin concerns. In this chapter, we'll cover some basic guidelines for selecting makeup for different skin types.

Makeup for oily skin

If you have oily skin, you'll want to choose makeup that is lightweight and oil-free, to help control shine and prevent breakouts. Look for products that are formulated for oily skin, such as:

- Oil-free foundation: An oil-free foundation will help to control shine and prevent breakouts. Look for a matte or semi-matte finish, as these are less likely to slide or melt off the skin.

- Powder: A setting powder or pressed powder can help to absorb excess oil and set your makeup in place.

- Oil-free blush: An oil-free blush will help to add a pop of color to your look without clogging pores or causing breakouts.

Makeup for dry skin

If you have dry skin, you'll want to choose makeup that is hydrating and nourishing, to help moisturize and protect the skin. Look for products that are formulated for dry skin, such as:

- Moisturizing foundation: A moisturizing foundation will help to hydrate and nourish the skin, while providing coverage and a natural, luminous finish.

- Cream eyeshadow: A cream eyeshadow will help to add color and dimension to your look without drying out the skin.

- Lip balm or lipstick: Choose a lip product that is moisturizing and nourishing, to help protect and hydrate the lips.

Makeup for combination skin

If you have combination skin, you'll want to choose makeup that is suitable for both your oily and dry areas. Look for products that are lightweight and oil-free, but still hydrating and nourishing, such as:

- Tinted moisturizer or BB cream: A tinted moisturizer or BB cream will help to even out your skin tone and provide a natural, luminous finish, without feeling heavy or greasy.

- Powder: A setting powder or pressed powder can help to absorb excess oil and set your makeup in place, without drying out the skin.

- Lip balm or lipstick: Choose a lip product that is moisturizing and nourishing, to help protect and hydrate the lips. Avoid matte formulas, as these can be drying and accentuate dryness.

By considering your skin type and selecting makeup that is suitable for your specific skin concerns, you'll be able to create a look that is flattering and enhances your natural beauty.

Chapter 17: Makeup for different seasons

Makeup looks can vary widely depending on the season. In the winter, you may want to choose makeup that is hydrating and nourishing, to help protect and moisturize the skin. In the summer, you may want to choose makeup that is lightweight and sweat-resistant, to help keep your skin looking fresh and cool. In this chapter, we'll cover some basic guidelines for selecting makeup for different seasons.

Makeup for winter

In the winter, you'll want to choose makeup that is hydrating and nourishing, to help protect and moisturize the skin. Look for products that are formulated for dry skin, such as:

- Moisturizing foundation: A moisturizing foundation will help to hydrate and nourish the skin, while providing coverage and a natural, luminous finish.

- Cream eyeshadow: A cream eyeshadow will help to add color and dimension to your look without drying out the skin.

- Lip balm or lipstick: Choose a lip product that is moisturizing and nourishing, to help protect and hydrate the lips.

Makeup for spring

In the spring, you'll want to choose makeup that is light and fresh, to help transition from the colder, drier winter months. Look for products that are sheer and luminous, such as:

- Tinted moisturizer or BB cream: A sheer, lightweight formula will help to even out your skin tone without looking heavy or cakey.

- Soft, neutral eyeshadow: A neutral eyeshadow palette will help to enhance your natural eye color and create a subtle, effortless look.

- Light, natural lipstick: Choose a light, natural shade of lipstick that is moisturizing and enhances your natural lip color.

Makeup for summer

In the summer, you'll want to choose makeup that is lightweight and sweat-resistant, to help keep your skin looking fresh and cool. Look for products that are formulated for oily or combination skin, such as:

- Oil-free foundation: An oil-free foundation will help to control shine and prevent breakouts, while feeling lightweight and comfortable on the skin.

- Powder: A setting powder or pressed powder can help to absorb excess oil and set your makeup in place, without feeling heavy or cakey.

- Oil-free blush: An oil-free blush will help to add a pop of color to your look without clogging pores or causing breakouts.

Makeup for fall

In the fall, you'll want to choose makeup that is rich and warm, to complement the changing leaves and cool, crisp air. Look for products that are highly pigmented and have a strong color payoff, such as:

- Full-coverage foundation: A full-coverage foundation will help to even out your skin tone and provide a flawless, airbrushed effect.

- Vibrant eyeshadow: A vibrant eyeshadow shade can add drama and impact to your look. Look for a shimmery or metallic shade to really make your eyes pop.

- Vibrant lipstick: A vibrant lipstick shade can add a pop of color to your look. Look for a shade that complements your skin tone and enhances your natural lip color.

By considering the season and selecting makeup that is suitable for the weather and your skin's needs, you'll be able to create a look that is flattering and enhances your natural beauty.

Chapter 18: Makeup for special occasions

Certain occasions call for a special kind of makeup look. Whether you're attending a wedding, a prom, or a fancy gala, you'll want to choose makeup that is appropriate for the occasion and enhances your natural beauty. In this chapter, we'll cover some basic guidelines for selecting makeup for special occasions.

Makeup for weddings

If you're attending a wedding, you'll want to choose makeup that is timeless and elegant, to complement the occasion. Look for products that are luminous and glowing, such as:

- Illuminating foundation: An illuminating foundation will help to add radiance and glow to the skin, while providing coverage and a natural finish.

- Soft, neutral eyeshadow: A neutral eyeshadow palette will help to enhance your natural eye color and create a subtle, effortless look.

- Lip balm or lipstick: Choose a lip product that is moisturizing and nourishing, to help protect and hydrate the lips. Avoid matte formulas, as these can be drying and accentuate the appearance of fine lines and wrinkles.

Makeup for prom

If you're attending prom, you'll want to choose makeup that is appropriate for your age and complements your dress and overall look. Look for products that are glamorous and glamorous, such as:

- Full-coverage foundation: A full-coverage foundation will help to even out your skin tone and provide a flawless, airbrushed effect.

- Vibrant eyeshadow: A vibrant eyeshadow shade can add drama and impact to your look. Look for a shimmery or metallic shade to really make your eyes pop.

- Vibrant lipstick: A vibrant lipstick shade can add a pop of color to your look. Look for a shade that complements your skin tone and enhances your natural lip color.

Makeup for fancy galas

If you're attending a fancy gala, you'll want to choose makeup that is sophisticated and polished, to complement the occasion. Look for products that are elegant and sophisticated, such as:

- Full-coverage foundation: A full-coverage foundation will help to even out your skin tone and provide a flawless, airbrushed effect.

- Soft, neutral eyeshadow: A neutral eyeshadow palette will help to enhance your natural eye color and create a subtle, effortless look.

- Lip balm or lipstick: Choose a lip product that is moisturizing and nourishing, to help protect and hydrate the lips. Avoid matte formulas, as these can be drying and accentuate the appearance of fine lines and wrinkles.

By considering the occasion and selecting makeup that is appropriate and enhances your natural beauty, you'll be able to create a look that is flattering and enhances your natural beauty.

Chapter 19: Makeup for everyday wear

For everyday wear, you'll want to choose makeup that is comfortable and easy to wear, while still enhancing your natural beauty. Look for products that are lightweight and natural-looking, such as:

Makeup for a natural look

If you prefer a natural, minimal makeup look, you'll want to choose products that are sheer and subtle, such as:

- Tinted moisturizer or BB cream: A sheer, lightweight formula will help to even out your skin tone without looking heavy or cakey.

- Soft, neutral eyeshadow: A neutral eyeshadow palette will help to enhance your natural eye color and create a subtle, effortless look.

- Lip balm or lipstick: Choose a lip product that is moisturizing and nourishing, to help protect and hydrate the lips.

Makeup for a polished look

If you prefer a polished, put-together makeup look, you'll want to choose products that are medium in coverage and intensity, such as:

- Medium-coverage foundation: A medium-coverage foundation will help to even out your skin tone and provide a natural, luminous finish.

- Soft, neutral eyeshadow: A neutral eyeshadow palette will help to enhance your natural eye color and create a subtle, effortless look.

- Lip balm or lipstick: Choose a lip product that is moisturizing and nourishing, to help protect and hydrate the lips.

By choosing makeup that is comfortable and easy to wear, you'll be able to create a look that is flattering and enhances your natural beauty, without taking up too much time or effort.

Chapter 20: Care about skin to look young for a long time

There are several things you can do to help your skin look young for a longer period of time:

1. Protect your skin from the sun: The sun's UV rays can damage your skin and cause premature aging, so it's important to protect your skin from the sun. Use a broad-spectrum sunscreen with an SPF of 30 or higher, and re-apply every two hours or after swimming or sweating.

2. Moisturize your skin: Moisturizing your skin can help to keep it hydrated and plump, which can help to reduce the appearance of fine lines and wrinkles. Choose a moisturizer that is suitable for your skin type and apply it daily.

3. Cleanse your skin: Proper cleansing can help to remove dirt, oil, and makeup from your skin, which can help to keep it looking fresh and healthy. Choose a gentle cleanser that is suitable for your skin type and use it twice a day.

4. Exfoliate your skin: Exfoliating your skin can help to remove dead skin cells, which can help to improve the appearance of your skin and give it a healthy glow. Choose an exfoliator that is suitable for your skin type and use it a few times a week.

5. Eat a healthy diet: A healthy diet that is rich in fruits, vegetables, and healthy fats can help to nourish your skin and keep it looking healthy and youthful. Avoid foods that are

high in sugar, salt, and unhealthy fats, as these can contribute to premature aging.

By taking good care of your skin and following these tips, you can help to keep your skin looking young and healthy for a longer period of time.

Chapter 21: Ten Steps Guide to Perfect Makeup

Follow these ten steps to achieve a perfect makeup look every time:

Step 1: Cleanse your skin

Before you start your makeup routine, it's important to cleanse your skin to remove any dirt, oil, and makeup from the day before. Choose a gentle cleanser that is suitable for your skin type and use it to wash your face, paying extra attention to the T-zone (forehead, nose, and chin).

Step 2: Tone your skin

After cleansing, use a toner to help balance your skin's pH and tighten your pores. Simply apply the toner to a cotton pad and swipe it over your face.

Step 3: Apply a moisturizer

Moisturizing your skin is an important step in your makeup routine, as it helps to hydrate and nourish your skin and create a smooth base for your makeup. Choose a moisturizer that is suitable for your skin type and apply it to your face, neck, and chest.

Step 4: Prime your skin

Applying a primer can help to smooth out your skin and create a perfect base for your makeup. Simply apply the primer to your face, paying extra attention to areas that tend to get oily or are prone to pores, such as the T-zone.

Step 5: Apply foundation

Foundation helps to even out your skin tone and create a smooth, uniform base for the rest of your makeup. Choose a foundation that is suitable for your skin type and apply it to your face using a brush, sponge, or your fingers.

Step 6: Conceal imperfections

Use a concealer to cover up any imperfections, such as blemishes, dark circles, or redness. Choose a concealer that is a shade lighter than your skin tone and apply it to the areas you want to cover, using a brush or your fingers to blend it in.

Step 7: Set your base with powder

Set your base with a setting powder to help your makeup stay in place and reduce shine. Simply dust the powder over your face using a brush or sponge, paying extra attention to the T-zone.

Step 8: Apply blush

Blush helps to add color and dimension to your face and can give you a healthy, rosy glow. Choose a blush that is suitable for your skin tone and apply it to the apples of your cheeks, blending upwards and outwards towards your temples.

Step 9: Define your eyes

Use eye makeup to define your eyes and create the desired look. This can include eyeshadow, liner, and mascara. Choose colors and formulas that are suitable for your eye shape and skin tone and apply them using brushes, sponges, or your fingers.

Step 10: Finish with lipstick or gloss

Finish your makeup look with a lip product, such as lipstick or gloss. Choose a shade that is suitable for your skin tone and apply it to your lips, using a brush or your fingers to blend it in.

By following these ten steps and using the right products and tools, you can achieve a perfect makeup look every time. Remember to customize your routine to suit your specific needs and preferences, and don't be afraid to experiment and try new things. With a little practice and patience, you'll be able to perfect your makeup routine and create a look that is beautiful and enhances your natural beauty.

Chapter 22: Special Makeup Applications

There are many special makeup applications that can help you create a unique and customized look.

These can include special effects makeup, airbrushing, and contouring. In this chapter, we'll cover some basic guidelines for these special makeup applications.

Special effects makeup

Special effects makeup is used to create illusions and special effects in movies, television, and theater. It can be used to create a wide range of looks, from scars and wounds to fantasy creatures and creatures. Special effects makeup can be complex and time-consuming to apply, and it often requires special techniques and materials.

Airbrushing

Airbrushing is a makeup application method that uses a compressor and airbrush gun to apply makeup to the skin. It is often used to create a smooth, even, and natural-looking finish, and it is especially effective for covering blemishes and imperfections. Airbrushing can be used to apply foundation, blush, and other makeup products, and it is often used in professional settings, such as photo shoots and fashion shows.

Contouring

Contouring is a makeup technique that involves using light and dark shades to create the illusion of depth and dimension on the face. It is often used to shape and define the facial features, such as the cheekbones, nose, and jawline. Contouring can be achieved using a variety of products, such as foundation, powder, and bronzer, and it requires precise application and blending to achieve a natural-looking result.

By learning these special makeup applications, you'll be able to create a wide range of looks and customize your makeup to suit your specific needs and preferences. With practice and patience, you'll be able to master these techniques and create beautiful, unique makeup looks.

Chapter 23: Skin Secrets

In this chapter, we'll share some secrets to help you achieve healthy, radiant skin. By following these tips and incorporating them into your skincare routine, you'll be able to nourish your skin and keep it looking beautiful and healthy.

Drink plenty of water

Drinking plenty of water can help to hydrate your skin and flush out toxins, which can help to keep your skin looking healthy and glowing. Aim to drink at least 8 cups of water per day, and more if you are active or live in a hot, dry climate.

Get enough sleep

Getting enough sleep is essential for healthy skin, as it gives your skin time to repair and regenerate. Aim for 7-9 hours of sleep per night and create a relaxing bedtime routine to help you wind down and fall asleep.

Eat a healthy diet

A healthy diet can help to nourish your skin and keep it looking healthy and youthful. Aim to eat plenty of fruits, vegetables, and healthy fats, and avoid foods that are high in sugar, salt, and unhealthy fats.

Exfoliate regularly

Exfoliating your skin can help to remove dead skin cells and reveal the healthy, radiant skin underneath. Choose an exfoliator that is suitable for your skin type and use it a few times a week, depending on your skin's needs.

Use skincare products that are suitable for your skin type

Using skincare products that are suitable for your skin type can help to nourish and protect your skin, and prevent irritation and breakouts. Choose products that are formulated for your specific skin concerns, such as acne, dryness, or aging, and follow the instructions for use.

By following these skin secrets and incorporating them into your skincare routine, you'll be able to nourish and protect your skin and keep it looking beautiful and healthy.

Conclusion

In conclusion, makeup can be a fun and creative way to enhance your natural beauty and express yourself. By learning about different makeup techniques, products, and tools, you'll be able to create a wide range of looks and customize your makeup to suit your specific needs and preferences.

By following the tips and guidelines outlined in this eBook, you'll be able to create beautiful, flawless makeup looks that enhance your natural beauty and make you feel confident and self-assured.

With practice and patience, you'll be able to master the art of makeup and create looks that are flattering, wearable, and appropriate for any occasion. Remember to take care of your skin and use makeup that is suitable for your skin type, and you'll be on your way to achieving beautiful, healthy, radiant skin.

Made in the USA
Las Vegas, NV
11 October 2023